COMPLETE GUIDE TO HEPATITIS

Comprehensive Insights, Symptoms, Prevention, Diagnosis, Treatment Strategies, Managing All Types, And Health Implications

DEHART HAIRSTON

DISCLAIMER

This book's content is only intended for general informative purposes. At the time of writing, the author has taken every precaution to guarantee that the material is correct and current. Nevertheless, the author disclaims all explicit and implicit representations and guarantees about the availability, appropriateness, correctness, completeness, and usefulness of the material on these pages.

Since the author is not a licensed medical practitioner, the material in this book shouldn't be interpreted as medical advice. Before making any modifications to their diet, exercise regimen, or medical treatment, readers are urged to speak with a licensed healthcare provider.

Moreover, the author has no connection to any of the businesses, organizations, or people that are discussed in this book. Any mentions of goods, services, businesses, or people are purely informative and do not indicate endorsement or suggestion.

This book's content is entirely dependent on the author's expertise, study, and comprehension of the topic. Despite having taken reasonable care to offer correct information, the author disclaims all liability for any mistakes or omissions in the material as well as for any losses, harm, or damages resulting from using the information.

It is recommended that readers use their own judgment and discretion when applying the knowledge in this book to their own situations. The use or implementation of any material in this book may result in unfavorable repercussions, directly or indirectly, for which the author assumes no liability.

By reading this book, you agree to release and hold the author harmless from any claims, losses, liabilities, costs, or expenditures resulting from or related to the use of the information you get from it.

Table of Contents

ABOUT THE BOOK

"Hepatitis" is more than simply a book; it's an extensive manual that may even save lives. It is critical to comprehend viral hepatitis in the modern world since it continues to pose a danger to public health. This book explores the subtleties of hepatitis in great detail, covering everything from the illness's history and symptoms to diagnosis, treatment, and prevention.

In addition to defining hepatitis and outlining its many forms, Chapter 1 establishes important background information about the condition's causes and risk factors. Anyone worried about their health or the health of a loved one must grasp these principles.

Next, Chapter 2 delves into the symptoms linked to hepatitis, explaining the similarities among the many forms as well as the differences that persist.

When it comes to knowing when to seek medical treatment, this chapter provides essential counsel that might save a life.

Chapter 3 provides a complete overview of the diagnostic methods that are essential to the management of hepatitis. This section provides readers with information on what to anticipate during diagnostic assessments, including blood tests, imaging methods, and liver biopsies.

Chapter 4 highlights the idea that prevention is always preferable to treatment by going over safe practices, vaccine alternatives, and lifestyle changes that may lower the risk of hepatitis. Through the use of the tactics discussed here, people may protect both themselves and their communities against this potentially crippling illness.

Specific forms of hepatitis are covered in detail in Chapters 5 through 9, along with information on how they are contracted, symptoms, available treatments, and long-term consequences on liver function. Not only is this information essential for those living with hepatitis, but it is also vital for medical professionals who want to improve their knowledge and treatment delivery.

Finally, Chapter 10 highlights the need to advocate and raise awareness. Readers may help tackle this hidden epidemic by actively engaging in public health programs and dispelling the stigma associated with hepatitis.

Essentially, "Hepatitis" is more than simply a book—it's a source of empowerment and information in the struggle against a major worldwide health issue. You can't afford to ignore this book since it is an essential resource for anybody seeking information, whether they are a patient, healthcare professional, or just an individual looking to learn more.

CHAPTER 1

Introduction To Hepatitis

The word "hepatitis" refers to an inflammation of the liver. Numerous things, such as viruses, alcoholism, autoimmune disorders, certain drugs, and poisons, might contribute to it. Maintaining liver health and avoiding major consequences need an understanding of hepatitis.

What Is Hepatitis?

The term "hepatitis" describes inflammation of the liver, an essential organ that processes nutrition, removes toxins from the blood, and makes key proteins. The liver's capacity to operate normally is hampered by inflammation, which may result in a variety of symptoms as well as possible problems.

Types Of Hepatitis (A, B, C, D, E)

distinct viruses may cause distinct forms of viral hepatitis. The hepatitis A, B, C, D, and E varieties are the most prevalent ones.

1. Hepatitis A: The usual way that an infected individual spreads the virus is via contaminated food, water, or intimate contact. It often only lasts a short while and doesn't progress to chronic liver disease. There is a vaccine available to protect against hepatitis A.

2. Hepatitis B: Blood, semen, or other bodily fluids contaminated with the virus may spread the disease to others. It may be chronic, last a lifetime, and perhaps result in severe liver damage, liver cancer, or cirrhosis, or it can be acute, lasting just a few weeks. Hepatitis B vaccination is also available.

3. Hepatitis C: The main way that the virus spreads is via coming into touch with contaminated blood, which often happens while exchanging needles or other injection supplies. It may result in acute or chronic hepatitis; over time, a chronic infection can progress to liver cirrhosis or liver cancer. Hepatitis C cannot be prevented, although it may be managed with antiviral drugs.

4. Hepatitis D: People who have previously had hepatitis B are the only ones who may get hepatitis D, commonly referred to as delta hepatitis. It may cause more serious liver damage and worsen the hepatitis B symptoms. Hepatitis D infection may be avoided with hepatitis B vaccine.

5. Hepatitis E: Drinking tainted water, especially in places with inadequate sanitation, is the main way that hepatitis E is transmitted. It causes acute hepatitis that usually goes away on its own, and its symptoms and duration are comparable to those of hepatitis A. As of right now, there is no readily accessible vaccination to prevent hepatitis E.

Causes and Risk Factors: Hepatitis has several causes depending on the kind of illness. Specific viruses cause viral hepatitis, but non-viral hepatitis may be brought on by exposure to chemicals, autoimmune disorders, alcoholism, or certain drugs.

Usually, viral hepatitis is transmitted by:

• Coming into contact with contaminated blood via blood transfusions or sharing of needles.

• Having sex with an infected individual.

• Eating or drinking tainted food or water.

• Vertical transmission of the infection from a woman sick to her infant child.

Causes And Risk Factors

• Taking part in high-risk activities like sharing needles or unprotected sex.

• Residing in or visiting places with high hepatitis infection rates and inadequate sanitation.

• Being immunocompromised as a result of HIV/AIDS or certain medical interventions.

• Operating in medical environments where contaminated blood or body fluids may be present.

Prevention and early identification of hepatitis depend on knowledge of its causes and risk factors. People may lower their chance of contracting hepatitis and safeguard their liver health by changing their lifestyle, getting vaccinated when it's available, avoiding sharing needles, and engaging in safe sexual practices.

CHAPTER 2

Understanding Hepatitis Symptoms

Common Symptoms Across Hepatitis Types

Whatever the form, hepatitis often presents with a few standard symptoms, thus identifying the warning signals is essential for prompt diagnosis and treatment. Typical symptoms include a general sensation of malaise and exhaustion, which may be incapacitating. This chronic fatigue may greatly interfere with day-to-day tasks and may not go away with rest.

Jaundice, which is marked by a yellowing of the skin and the whites of the eyes, is another common symptom. A yellow pigment called bilirubin accumulates in the circulation and causes jaundice, which is indicative of liver failure. In addition to jaundice, some people may have pale stools and dark urine, which are signs of abnormal liver function.

Typical gastrointestinal symptoms of hepatitis include nausea and vomiting. People may lose their appetite, which might result in inadvertent weight loss. Moreover, inflammation and enlargement of the liver might result in pain or discomfort in the abdomen, especially in the upper right quadrant.

In addition to low-grade fever, some hepatitis patients may also have flu-like symptoms such as joint and muscular discomfort. The kind of hepatitis and personal health conditions might affect the strength and duration of these symptoms.

Variations In Symptoms Based On Hepatitis Type

Some differences set each form of hepatitis apart, even if certain symptoms are common to all of them. Compared to other forms, hepatitis A usually exhibits milder symptoms at first. People with hepatitis A sometimes don't even show any symptoms, particularly in young children. When symptoms do appear, they often consist of jaundice, exhaustion, nausea, and vomiting as well as stomach discomfort.

Both acute and chronic infections may result from hepatitis B and C, with acute infections sometimes showing no symptoms at all or very mild signs that resemble those of hepatitis A. On the other hand, if untreated, persistent hepatitis B and C infections might eventually cause more serious liver damage. Chronic symptoms of hepatitis B and C might include jaundice, dark urine, lethargy, and stomach discomfort. Furthermore, liver cirrhosis and liver cancer are two more severe side effects of chronic hepatitis.

Though less frequent, hepatitis D and E might make hepatitis B and A symptoms worse, respectively.

Hepatitis D may lead to more severe liver damage and often exclusively affects those who have previously had hepatitis B. Although hepatitis E usually resolves on its own, there are situations where it might progress to fulminant hepatitis, a potentially fatal illness, particularly in pregnant women.

When To Seek Medical Attention

Effective hepatitis management depends on knowing when to get medical help. It is best to get medical attention right once if you have symptoms like chronic exhaustion, jaundice, stomach discomfort, or black urine. Furthermore, it's critical to be tested for hepatitis if you have participated in risky activities like sharing needles or unprotected sexual activity, or if you have been exposed to someone who has the virus.

If you have severe symptoms, such as severe stomach discomfort, disorientation, or bleeding tendencies, get help right away since these might be signs of acute liver failure, a life-threatening condition that has to be treated quickly.

For people who are at high risk, such as those who have used intravenous drugs in the past, have had many sexual partners, or are healthcare professionals who have come into contact with blood products, routine hepatitis screening is advised. Early identification via screening lowers the risk of complications from hepatitis and enables prompt treatments. Do not hesitate to call your healthcare practitioner for an examination and proper therapy if you believe you may have been exposed to hepatitis or if you are exhibiting symptoms indicative of the illness.

CHAPTER 3

Diagnostic Procedures

Blood Tests For Hepatitis Markers

Blood tests are essential for identifying hepatitis and aiding medical professionals in comprehending the kind, intensity, and course of the illness. The main purpose of these tests is to find certain markers that point to viral hepatitis infections. The A, B, and C hepatitis viruses are the most prevalent ones and have different symptoms.

IgM antibodies generated during the acute stage of infection are used to identify the hepatitis A virus (HAV). After exposure, these antibodies often start to show up two to four weeks later and start to wane six months later. The main indicator of both acute and chronic hepatitis B infection is hepatitis B surface antigen (HBsAg).

It may last for weeks or months and is a sign that the virus is in the bloodstream. Furthermore, the presence of hepatitis B surface antibodies (anti-HBs) and hepatitis B core antibodies (anti-HBc) provides light on the infection's stage and immunity level.

Testing for the hepatitis C virus (HCV) entails looking for antibodies to the virus. To confirm acute infection, however, a different test for HCV RNA (genetic material) could be required since antibodies take time to develop. When taken as a whole, these blood tests provide a complete picture of the hepatitis infection, which may help with treatment choices and disease progression tracking.

Imaging Tests (Ultrasound, MRI, CT Scan)

Imaging studies are essential for determining the condition of the liver and spotting hepatitis-related problems.

Imaging tests such as ultrasound, MRI, and CT scans are often used to view the liver, identify anomalies, and assess the degree of liver damage.

Because ultrasound is affordable, safe, and easy to use, it is often the first imaging modality used. Healthcare professionals may evaluate the liver's size, texture, and existence of lesions or fluid buildup by using the real-time pictures it offers. Furthermore, cirrhosis, portal hypertension, and hepatocellular carcinoma (liver cancer) may all be detected by ultrasonography.

The detection of issues connected to hepatitis may be aided by the more comprehensive pictures of the liver and surrounding structures provided by MRI and CT studies. Because MRI doesn't utilize ionizing radiation and offers improved soft tissue contrast, it's very helpful for assessing liver function and finding tiny lesions. Conversely, bigger lesions, vascular anomalies, and indications of advanced liver disease are best detected by CT scans.

Healthcare professionals can effectively diagnose hepatitis, track the disease's course, and customize treatment plans for each patient by integrating data from imaging examinations and blood testing.

Liver Biopsy: What To Expect

By taking a tiny sample of liver tissue for microscopic analysis, a liver biopsy operation may provide important information about the condition of the liver, the severity of the illness, and how well a therapy is working. Even while it can seem scary, knowing what to anticipate helps allay fears and guarantee a positive encounter.

Your healthcare professional will go over the purpose, dangers, and advantages of the biopsy with you before the operation. To lessen the chance of bleeding, you could be instructed to stop taking certain drugs, such as blood thinners. To reduce pain, local anesthetic is usually used during the surgery.

You will lie on your side or back during the biopsy, and the medical professional will use ultrasound or CT imaging to help them find the best location for tissue collection. The liver is then punctured with a tiny needle to extract a sample of tissue. During the needle insertion, you can feel pressure or experience a momentary pain.

You will be kept under observation for a few hours after the biopsy to make sure there are no unanticipated problems, including discomfort or bleeding. Mild tenderness at the biopsy site is common and is often treatable with over-the-counter pain medication. Your healthcare professional will talk with you about the biopsy results, which are usually available in a week.

A liver biopsy yields important data that may be used to monitor medication response, evaluate the course of the illness, and guide treatment options. Although there are some hazards involved, such as bleeding or infection, these are uncommon and may be reduced by closely adhering to pre- and post-procedure instructions. In general, liver biopsy is a reliable and crucial treatment option for liver disease and hepatitis.

CHAPTER 4

Hepatitis Prevention

Vaccination Against Hepatitis A And B

One of the best defenses against hepatitis, especially hepatitis A and B, is vaccination. While hepatitis B is primarily disseminated by contact with infected blood or body fluids, hepatitis A is typically transferred via contaminated food or water. Both vaccinations are readily accessible, safe, and strongly advised for anyone who may be exposed.

Typically, two doses of the hepatitis A vaccination are administered, spaced six to twelve months apart. Travelers visiting areas with a high prevalence of hepatitis A, those with chronic liver illness, men who have sex with males, and illegal drug users may consider it since it offers long-term protection against the infection.

By receiving a vaccination, you lessen the transmission of the virus by protecting others as well as strengthening community immunity.

Comparably, depending on the brand, the hepatitis B vaccination is given in a series of three or four doses. It is advised for newborns, kids, teenagers, and adults who are at risk of contracting hepatitis B, as well as healthcare professionals, those who have had many sexual partners, and those who have certain medical issues. By encouraging the production of antibodies by the immune system against the hepatitis B virus, the vaccination confers immunity and guards against infection.

It's crucial to understand that vaccinations only stop new infections from happening; they do not cure pre-existing hepatitis illnesses. Consequently, vaccination is essential before any viral exposure. Furthermore, the majority of individuals are safe to have both vaccinations and the few adverse effects, which usually go away on their own, include minor fever or injection site discomfort.

For certain people, particularly those with compromised immune systems or long-term exposure to hepatitis risk factors, regular booster doses may be advised. All things considered, vaccination against hepatitis A and B is an important preventative measure against these potentially dangerous and fatal illnesses, providing long-term health advantages as well as mental peace of mind.

Safe Practices To Prevent Hepatitis Transmission

Adopting safe procedures is crucial for stopping the spread of hepatitis viruses, in addition to immunization. Hepatitis B, C, and D are mostly transferred by contact with contaminated blood or body fluids, while hepatitis A and E are mainly disseminated by contaminated food or water. You may drastically lower your chance of getting these infections by adhering to a few easy-to-follow yet powerful instructions.

Primarily, maintaining proper cleanliness is essential for halting the spread of hepatitis. This involves cleaning your hands well with soap and water after using the toilet, before consuming or preparing food, and after coming into contact with surfaces or things that may be contaminated. Maintaining good hand hygiene lowers the possibility of spreading viruses to other people as well as to yourself by helping to eliminate any that may be on your hands.

Furthermore, the likelihood of contracting hepatitis may be significantly reduced by abstaining from dangerous activities. This includes being tested for hepatitis often if you participate in high-risk activities, avoiding sharing needles or other drug paraphernalia, and practicing safe sex by using condoms consistently and appropriately. Hepatitis A and E infections may also be avoided by abstaining from tainted food and water, particularly in places with inadequate sanitation.

Healthcare professionals and other individuals at occupational risk of hepatitis exposure must take the recommended safeguards. This entails disposing of sharps and other potentially contaminated objects carefully as well as using the proper personal protective equipment, including gloves, masks, and gowns while handling blood or bodily fluids. Healthcare facilities may reduce the chance of hepatitis transmission to patients and staff by putting these safeguards in place.

Another important factor in stopping the spread of hepatitis is education. By educating people on how infections spread and how to avoid them, people will be better equipped to make choices about how to keep themselves and others safe. Healthcare professionals, educational initiatives, and community-based programs may all help spread correct information and encourage healthy lifestyle choices.

You can help prevent the spread of hepatitis and make your community a safer and healthier place for everyone by incorporating these safe practices into your everyday life and advocating for them.

Lifestyle Changes For Hepatitis Risk Reduction

Aside from immunization and safe practices, altering one's lifestyle may help lower the chance of contracting hepatitis and improve liver health in general. Several lifestyle choices, including drug and alcohol abuse, poor eating habits, and excessive alcohol use, may worsen the symptoms of hepatitis and raise the risk of liver damage.

You may lessen the damage that hepatitis does to your health and safeguard your liver by changing to healthy habits.

Reducing or quitting alcohol completely is one of the biggest lifestyle adjustments you can make to lower your risk of hepatitis. Particularly in those with viral hepatitis, excessive alcohol use may lead to liver inflammation, cirrhosis, and other severe liver illnesses. You may save your liver and reduce the chance of complications from hepatitis by reducing your alcohol use or getting help for alcoholism.

In a similar vein, abstaining from illegal drug use—especially injectable drug use—is crucial for lowering the risk of hepatitis. Sharing needles or other drug paraphernalia raises the chance of contracting other bloodborne illnesses like hepatitis B, C, and D considerably. Seeking therapy and support services may help you overcome drug addiction and safeguard your health if you suffer from it.

A balanced diet and consistent exercise may also promote liver health and lower the risk of liver disease. Whole grains, lean meats, fruits, and vegetables all contribute to a balanced diet that is full of minerals and antioxidants that promote liver function and lower inflammation. Frequent exercise improves liver function overall, lowers cholesterol, and helps people maintain a healthy weight.

For liver health and hepatitis risk reduction, it's also critical to manage other chronic health issues including obesity, diabetes, and hypertension. These illnesses may worsen liver damage and raise the possibility of complications from hepatitis. You may safeguard your liver and general health by collaborating with your healthcare professional to treat these problems via medication, lifestyle modifications, and routine monitoring.

In conclusion, modifying one's lifestyle to include less alcohol intake, abstaining from illegal drug use, maintaining regular exercise and diet, and treating long-term medical issues may all help lower the chance of contracting hepatitis and improve liver function. You may take proactive measures to protect yourself against hepatitis and have a happier, happier life by giving priority to certain lifestyle variables.

CHAPTER 5

Hepatitis A: The Basics

Transmission Routes And Risk Factors

The hepatitis A virus (HAV) is the extremely contagious cause of hepatitis A, often known as infectious hepatitis. Preventing its spread requires an understanding of how it spreads and the variables that raise the risk of transmission.

The main way that hepatitis A is spread is via eating or drinking infected food or water. The virus may readily contaminate food or water supplies if basic sanitation procedures are not followed. It is often detected in the feces of infected persons. Close physical contact with an infected individual may also aid in transmission, such as while engaging in sexual activity or tending to a sick person.

Hepatitis A risk is increased by certain variables. Travelers visiting areas with inadequate sanitation and hygiene standards are at a higher risk of contracting the virus. In a similar vein, those who engage in high-risk activities like intravenous drug use or several sexual partners are more likely to get infected. Additionally, there is an increased risk of contracting hepatitis A in those who live in crowded or unhygienic environments.

Reducing the risk of hepatitis A transmission requires the use of preventative measures. The virus may be stopped from spreading by practicing good hand hygiene, which includes often washing your hands with soap and water. Furthermore, it is important to follow safe food and water hygiene practices, such as abstaining from uncooked shellfish and only drinking clean, purified water, particularly while visiting regions where hepatitis A is common. It is also advised that those who are at risk of infection—such as visitors to areas where hepatitis A is prevalent and members of certain high-risk groups—vaccinate against the virus.

People may take preventative measures to shield themselves and others from hepatitis A by being aware of the risk factors and channels of transmission.

Symptoms And Duration Of Illness

Early diagnosis and timely medical intervention are contingent upon the ability to identify the signs of hepatitis A. After being exposed to the virus, symptoms usually start to show up two to six weeks later, but in rare circumstances, they could take up to 50 days. Effective management of sickness may be facilitated by an understanding of the length of the illness and the course of symptoms.

Hepatitis A may cause a range of symptoms, from minor to severe, such as exhaustion, nausea, vomiting, stomach discomfort, and appetite loss. Jaundice, which is characterized by pale feces, dark urine, and yellowing of the skin and eyes, may also affect certain people. The immunological reaction and general health state of the person might affect the degree and duration of symptoms.

Hepatitis A is often a self-limiting disease, meaning that it goes away on its own without the need for special medical care. But the sickness may last anywhere from a few weeks to several months, and some people may continue to feel tired and unwell long after the acute phase has ended. Seeking medical treatment is crucial for anyone suspected of having hepatitis A to get a thorough diagnosis and supportive therapy.

People with hepatitis A should avoid alcohol and some drugs that might further strain their liver during the acute phase of the disease and instead focus on rest.

Sustaining proper hydration and nourishment is crucial for bolstering the immune system and expediting the healing process. Hospitalization could be required in extreme situations to monitor liver function and provide intravenous fluids or other supportive care.

To get the right medical attention and successfully treat hepatitis A, people must be aware of the illness's symptoms and duration. People may lessen the effects of hepatitis A on their health and well-being by being aware of the symptoms and acting promptly to treat them.

Treatment Options And Prognosis

Hepatitis A does not yet have a particular therapy, but managing symptoms and providing supportive care is crucial for encouraging recovery and avoiding consequences. Making educated healthcare choices may be facilitated by knowledge about the prognosis and current treatment options for hepatitis A.

The goals of supportive treatment for hepatitis A include liver function preservation and symptom relief. To aid the body in healing from the illness, supportive treatment should include rest, plenty of water, and a healthy diet. Hospitalization could be required in extreme situations to monitor liver function and provide intravenous fluids or other supportive care.

Apart from receiving supportive treatment, it is essential to refrain from drugs like alcohol and certain medicines that may exacerbate liver damage to facilitate hepatitis A recovery. To guarantee a full recovery from hepatitis A, patients should also adhere to the advice of their medical professional about follow-up treatment and liver function monitoring.

The majority of people with hepatitis A recover fully from the virus in a matter of weeks to months, making the prognosis typically optimistic. Hepatitis A may, however, in rare instances have consequences like abrupt liver failure, particularly in elderly people or those with underlying liver disease. To avoid difficulties and guarantee a good result, early identification, and timely medical intervention are crucial.

Immunization against hepatitis A is advised for anyone who may be exposed, such as visitors to areas where the disease is prevalent and members of certain high-risk populations. The vaccination is quite successful at avoiding infection. By being aware of the prognosis and available treatments for hepatitis A, people may take preventative measures to avoid infection and efficiently treat the illness in case it manifests.

CHAPTER 6

Hepatitis B: What You Need To Know

Modes Of Transmission And Prevention

The main ailment of hepatitis B is a viral infection of the liver, and prevention requires knowledge of how the illness spreads. There are a few ways the virus may spread, but coming into touch with contaminated blood, semen, or other body fluids is the most typical one. Unprotected sexual contact, sharing needles or other drug paraphernalia, or mother-to-child transmission after delivery may all lead to this. Sharing personal objects like toothbrushes or razors that may have come into touch with contaminated blood may also transmit hepatitis B.

Several crucial tactics are needed to stop the spread of hepatitis B. First and foremost, immunization has a very high rate of illness prevention. All newborns and people who may be at higher risk of exposure are advised to get the hepatitis B vaccination, which is normally given in a series of injections. Important preventative steps include sharing needles or other drug-related equipment and practicing safe intercourse by using condoms. In addition, minimizing the risk of transmission in clinical settings is achieved by making sure that healthcare institutions adhere to stringent infection control standards, such as properly sanitizing medical equipment and utilizing disposable needles.

Efforts to prevent this also must prioritize education and awareness. People may take proactive measures to safeguard others and themselves by being aware of the transmission mechanisms of hepatitis B and the precautions that can be taken to lower the risk of infection. This entails being aware of the value of immunization, engaging in safe behavior, and getting help if you get infected with the virus.

Acute Vs. Chronic Hepatitis B

There are two main types of hepatitis B infection manifestations: acute and chronic. The phrase "acute hepatitis B" describes an illness that usually lasts a few weeks to many months. As their immune systems react to the virus during this period, people may suffer symptoms including exhaustion, nausea, jaundice, stomach discomfort, and black urine. The majority of individuals who have acute hepatitis B can get rid of the virus from their systems without any long-term effects.

Hepatitis B infection, however, may sometimes become chronic. When the virus stays in the body for six months or more, it may cause chronic hepatitis B. Chronic hepatitis B, in contrast to acute infection, may cause more severe health problems, such as cirrhosis, liver damage, and an elevated risk of liver cancer. Early testing and monitoring are crucial for avoiding consequences since many patients with chronic hepatitis B may not show any symptoms for years or even decades.

Individual differences in the course of acute to chronic hepatitis B include age, immunological response, and underlying medical problems. Some people can get rid of the virus on their own, while others can have a persistent infection that has to be treated medically for the rest of their lives.

Treatment Options And Management Strategies

The goals of hepatitis B treatment are to contain the infection, avoid liver damage, and lower the chance of complications.

Depending on the illness stage and the kind of infection (chronic or acute), several treatment options are available.

Treatment for acute hepatitis B often consists of symptom relief and supportive measures. This might include getting enough rest, drinking enough of water, and using over-the-counter painkillers to ease discomfort. Generally, the virus may be eliminated by the immune system without the need for specialized antiviral medication.

On the other hand, continual medical care is necessary for chronic hepatitis B to suppress the virus and avoid liver damage. The cornerstone of care for persistent infections is the use of antiviral drugs, of which several varieties impede viral reproduction. These drugs may lessen the risk of cirrhosis and liver cancer, lessen inflammation in the liver, and enhance liver function in general.

For the treatment of chronic hepatitis B, lifestyle changes are as important as antiviral medication. This includes abstaining from alcohol, which may aggravate liver disease, keeping up a nutritious diet, getting regular exercise, and avoiding drugs that might be hazardous to the liver. It's also critical to do routine imaging examinations and blood tests to evaluate liver function and identify any issues early.

Liver transplantation could be required for some people with advanced liver disease or its consequences, such as cirrhosis or liver cancer. For patients who have end-stage liver disease, this may be a life-saving procedure that entails surgically substituting a healthy donor liver for the diseased liver.

All things considered, managing and treating hepatitis B necessitates a thorough strategy that takes into account the viral infection itself as well as any possible long-term effects. Hepatitis B patients can control their illness and lower their risk of complications by combining antiviral medication with lifestyle changes and routine monitoring.

CHAPTER 7

Hepatitis C: Understanding The Silent Epidemic

Transmission Routes And High-Risk Populations

Preventing the spread of hepatitis C requires an understanding of how the virus spreads. Contact with contaminated blood is the main way that hepatitis C is transmitted. This may occur in several ways, including sharing needles or injecting equipment, having a tattoo or piercing using non-sterilized equipment, and receiving blood transfusions before 1992, when screening techniques were less sophisticated. Sexual intercourse may also spread hepatitis C, however, the danger is not as great as it is with other transmission pathways.

Hepatitis C is more likely to infect certain groups. Individuals who inject drugs are disproportionately impacted, especially those who share needles. A significant percentage of newly diagnosed cases of hepatitis C are related to this group. Those who had organ transplants or blood transfusions before the strict screening protocols being put in place are likewise vulnerable. Another high-risk category includes healthcare personnel who could unintentionally stab themselves with needles and come into touch with contaminated blood. It is also more likely for the offspring of hepatitis C-positive moms to get the disease.

Reducing the spread of hepatitis C requires preventive actions. New infections may be avoided by encouraging drug users to inject drugs more safely, encouraging the use of sterile needles and supplies, and raising awareness of the significance of safe sexual behaviors.

Furthermore, limiting the danger of infection via organ transplants and blood donations requires the implementation of stringent screening measures. The spread of hepatitis C must be stopped by public health programs that educate at-risk groups and provide them access to testing and treatment.

The Link Between Hepatitis C And Liver Disease

Comprehending the relationship between hepatitis C and liver disease is crucial since it is a primary cause of liver disease globally. Over time, the hepatitis C virus infection may cause liver damage by inducing inflammation in the liver. Damage of this kind may lead to more serious ailments including liver cancer, cirrhosis, and fibrosis.

When there is chronic inflammation, the liver tissue scars and develops fibrosis. When fibrosis worsens, it may result in cirrhosis, a condition marked by severe scarring that affects liver function. The likelihood of complications including liver failure and portal hypertension, which may have detrimental effects on general health, is greatly increased by cirrhosis.

Liver cancer may sometimes result from a hepatitis C infection, especially in those with severe liver disease. In patients with hepatitis C, hepatocellular carcinoma (HCC) is the most prevalent form of liver cancer. People with cirrhosis have an increased chance of developing HCC, which emphasizes the need to treat and diagnose hepatitis C early to stop the disease's development.

Controlling the hepatitis C virus is crucial for stopping the advancement of liver damage. The goals of treatment are to lessen liver inflammation, stop the virus from spreading, and stop additional liver damage. Early detection and treatment may greatly enhance results and lower the chance of side effects like liver cancer and cirrhosis. It is essential for people with hepatitis C to regularly evaluate their liver function using imaging examinations and blood tests to identify any early warning signals of the disease's development and take appropriate action.

Advances In Hepatitis C Treatment And Cure

Significant progress has been achieved in the treatment of hepatitis C in recent years, giving many infected people hope for a recovery. Interferon-based regimens were the mainstay of conventional hepatitis C treatment choices, but they often had serious side effects and were not very effective. Nonetheless, the development of direct-acting antiviral (DAA) drugs has completely changed how hepatitis C is treated.

DAA drugs stop the hepatitis C virus from replicating and spreading within the body by focusing on certain stages of the virus's reproduction cycle. In most situations, these drugs have cure rates higher than 95%, demonstrating their excellent effectiveness. DAA regimens also often have fewer adverse effects and are more tolerated than previous treatment methods.

The therapeutic landscape for hepatitis C has changed significantly with the introduction of highly effective and well-tolerated DAA medicines. Regardless of the virus's genotype or the existence of liver cirrhosis, these drugs provide most hepatitis C patients with a chance of recovery. Additionally, the length of treatment has been drastically reduced; current DAA regimens only call for 8 to 12 weeks of medication.

Many regions of the globe now have better access to hepatitis C treatment because of initiatives to lower the cost of medications and raise public knowledge of the significance of screening and treatment. Accessibility issues persist, nevertheless, especially in low- and middle-income nations where resources may be few. It is imperative to tackle these obstacles through activism, legislative modifications, and global cooperation to guarantee that everyone impacted by hepatitis C may get treatment that can save lives.

CHAPTER 8

Living With Hepatitis: Tips For Management

Dietary Recommendations For Liver Health

For those with hepatitis, eating a balanced diet is essential since it affects liver function and general health. In addition to supporting liver regeneration, a balanced diet may aid with discomfort relief and inflammation reduction. Here are some nutritional suggestions to think about:

1. **Reduce Your Alcohol Consumption:** Alcohol may worsen liver disease since it is metabolized by the liver. It's essential to either completely give up alcohol or cut down on usage.

2. **Emphasis on healthy Foods:** Make sure your diet includes an abundance of fruits, vegetables, healthy grains, and lean meats. These meals promote liver

function and general health because they are high in fiber, antioxidants, and vital minerals.

3. Limit Sodium Intake: Consuming too much sodium may cause edema and fluid retention, which can exacerbate liver problems. Choose low-sodium substitutes and stay away from processed meals that are heavy in salt.

4. Select Good Fats: Go for unsaturated fats, which are present in foods like avocados, nuts, seeds, and fatty fish like mackerel and salmon. These fats promote heart health and help lower inflammation.

5. Moderate Protein Intake: Although too much protein might cause liver strain, it is necessary for both general health and muscle regeneration. Pick modest quantities of lean protein sources including fish, chicken, tofu, and lentils.

6. Drink Plenty of Water: Both liver function and general health depend on drinking enough water. Try to avoid sugary drinks and drink plenty of water throughout the day.

7. Think About vitamins: Milk thistle, vitamin D, and vitamin E are a few vitamins that some hepatitis patients may find helpful. But, before beginning any new supplement regimen, it's important to speak with a healthcare professional since certain supplements may worsen liver problems or interfere with prescription drugs.

People with hepatitis may improve their general health and liver health, which will improve their quality of life, by adhering to these dietary guidelines.

Medication Adherence And Monitoring

Effective hepatitis management requires taking prescription drugs as directed and being checked on often. Effective pharmaceutical treatment may lessen symptoms, stop complications, and decrease the course of the illness. What you should know about monitoring and adherence to medicine is as follows:

1. Adhere to Your Treatment Plan: It's critical that you take your meds as directed by your physician. Medication resistance and decreased treatment efficacy might result from missing or adjusting dosages.

2. Set Reminders: To help you remember to take your meds on time, use pill organizers, alarm clocks, or smartphone applications. To get the best outcomes possible, consistency is essential.

3. Talk to Your Healthcare Team: Don't be afraid to contact your healthcare provider if you have any adverse effects or are having trouble following your treatment plan.

They may give advice, change your prescription if needed, or recommend other options for help.

4. Attend Check-ups regularly: Monitoring liver function, determining the effectiveness of medication, and identifying any possible consequences early on all depend on regular monitoring. Make sure you show up for all of your doctor's visits on time, and do any required tests exactly as directed.

5. Track Your Progress: Keep a log of the drugs you take, the amounts you take, and any adverse effects or symptoms you encounter. Together with your healthcare practitioner, you may use this information to monitor your progress and decide on an appropriate treatment strategy.

Hepatitis patients may enhance their general health and well-being and maximize treatment success by emphasizing drug adherence and routine monitoring.

Coping Strategies And Support Resources

Hepatitis may cause physical discomfort, psychological stress, and lifestyle changes, among other difficulties. People may improve their quality of life and traverse these problems with the use of coping mechanisms and support systems. The following are some tactics and sources to think about:

1. Seek Emotional Support: It may be emotionally draining to have a chronic illness such as hepatitis. Think about joining an online or in-person support group where you can talk to others going through similar things. Vital emotional support may also be obtained by speaking with friends, family, or a mental health professional.

2. Use stress-reduction strategies: Stress may worsen symptoms and hurt general health. To encourage relaxation and mental health, include stress-reduction practices like yoga, tai chi, deep breathing exercises, mindfulness, and meditation in your daily routine.

3. Keep Yourself Educated: Information empowers. Learn about the signs and symptoms of hepatitis, as well as available treatments and self-care techniques. You'll feel more in control and be better able to make health-related choices if you know what your condition is like.

4. Keep a Positive Attitude: Although having hepatitis may be difficult, keeping a positive outlook can greatly impact how you manage the illness. Pay attention to what you can manage, acknowledge and appreciate little things in life, and practice thankfulness every day.

5. Access Assistance Services: Make use of the resources that are available to you in terms of assistance, including patient advocacy groups, hotlines, and instructional materials. These sites may provide helpful information, help navigating healthcare systems, and emotional support specifically designed for hepatitis patients.

People with hepatitis may successfully manage their disease, improve their quality of life, and flourish despite any problems they may encounter by putting coping methods into practice and making use of support services.

CHAPTER 9

Hepatitis And Liver Health

Long-Term Effects Of Hepatitis On The Liver

Hepatitis may have serious long-term consequences on the liver, regardless of whether it is brought on by a virus like hepatitis B or hepatitis C or by other factors like heavy alcohol usage. It is essential to comprehend these impacts to manage and avoid issues.

Liver inflammation is one of the main chronic consequences of hepatitis on the liver. Hepatitis virus infection of the liver causes inflammation by inducing an immunological response. Acute inflammation is the body's normal reaction to an infection or injury, but persistent inflammation may harm liver cells and compromise liver function over time.

Liver fibrosis, a disorder marked by a buildup of scar tissue in the liver, may develop from chronic hepatitis. Liver cirrhosis is a late stage of liver scarring that may develop from hepatic fibrosis over time. When cirrhosis occurs, the liver loses its capacity to function normally and becomes lumpy and hard. Numerous problems, such as portal hypertension, ascites (abdominal fluid accumulation), hepatic encephalopathy (impairing of brain function), and liver failure, may arise from this.

Additionally, the chance of developing liver cancer is increased by chronic hepatitis infection, especially with the Hepatitis B and Hepatitis C viruses. Hepatocellular carcinoma (HCC) is the most prevalent kind of liver cancer, and it may grow over time as a result of the ongoing inflammation and damage to liver cells produced by these viruses. While hepatitis C is a significant cause of liver cancer in affluent nations, hepatitis B is the primary cause of liver cancer globally.

Ongoing monitoring and therapy are necessary to manage the liver's long-term consequences of hepatitis. To evaluate liver health and identify any indications of disease development, this may include routine liver function tests, imaging tests (such as MRIs or ultrasounds), and liver biopsies. In addition, people with chronic hepatitis B or C may be offered antiviral medicines to limit viral replication and minimize inflammation of the liver.

Liver Cirrhosis And Liver Cancer Risk

A major side effect of long-term liver illness, such as a persistent hepatitis infection, is liver cirrhosis, which raises the chance of developing liver cancer. For early identification and management, it is important to comprehend the connection between cirrhosis and the risk of liver cancer.

As was previously established, the gradual buildup of scar tissue in the liver causes liver cirrhosis, which compromises liver function. Numerous conditions may lead to cirrhosis, such as autoimmune liver disorders, excessive alcohol use, chronic hepatitis B or C infection, and non-alcoholic fatty liver disease (NAFLD).

The formation of regenerating nodules inside the injured liver tissue is one of the main reasons connecting cirrhosis to the risk of liver cancer. In reaction to liver damage, these nodules are regions of continuous cell growth and regeneration. Regenerative nodules are initially benign, but with time they may develop into malignant tumors due to genetic abnormalities.

Those who have cirrhosis are more at risk for liver cancer. Research indicates that those with cirrhosis have a markedly increased yearly risk of developing liver cancer in comparison to those without the condition. While intrahepatic cholangiocarcinoma is one of the rarer forms of liver cancer, hepatocellular carcinoma (HCC) is the most prevalent kind linked with cirrhosis.

Patients with cirrhosis should undergo routine monitoring for liver cancer to identify tumors at an early stage that may be treatable. This usually includes blood tests to evaluate liver function and tumor indicators, as well as imaging examinations like ultrasounds, CT scans, or MRIs, done every six months.

In addition to monitoring, managing modifiable risk factors including alcohol use and hepatitis virus infection is a key component of attempts to prevent liver cancer in people with cirrhosis. Depending on the stage and severity of the disease, treatment options for liver cancer may include liver transplantation, surgical resection, locoregional therapies (such as transarterial chemoembolization or radiofrequency ablation), and systemic therapies (such as immunotherapy or targeted therapies).

Importance Of Regular Liver Health Check-Ups

For the early diagnosis and treatment of liver illness, especially complications from hepatitis, routine liver health examinations are essential. Healthcare professionals can monitor liver function, evaluate the course of the illness, and take quick action to stop more liver damage thanks to these checkups.

A liver health check-up may include several tests to assess liver function and look for any indications of liver disease. These examinations often consist of:

1. Tests for liver function (LFTs): These blood tests quantify the amounts of proteins and enzymes that show how well the liver is working.

Results from an abnormal LFT test might indicate inflammation, damage, or malfunctioning of the liver.

2. Hepatitis B and C virus screening: In particular, for those who are more susceptible to infection, screening tests for these two viruses may be advised. Timely intervention and therapy to avoid liver damage are made possible by early identification of viral hepatitis.

3. Imaging studies: The liver may be seen and any anomalies, such as liver enlargement, fatty liver disease, or liver tumors, can be found using imaging methods including ultrasonography, CT scans, or MRIs.

4. Liver biopsy: A liver biopsy is a procedure that may sometimes be used to take a little sample of liver tissue for microscopic analysis. This process aids in the diagnosis of liver disorders, evaluation of the extent of liver damage, and direction of therapeutic choices.

People who have risk factors for liver disease, such as a history of liver disease in their family, excessive alcohol intake, obesity, diabetes, or chronic hepatitis infection, should have regular liver health examinations. Early detection of liver issues allows medical professionals to better manage patients' long-term health by preventing or delaying the advancement of liver disease and implementing appropriate therapies, such as medication, lifestyle changes, or surgical procedures.

Preserving liver health and avoiding consequences from hepatitis and other liver illnesses require making routine liver health examinations a priority. These examinations enable people to take preventative measures to safeguard their liver and general health, which eventually improves health and quality of life.

CHAPTER 10

Spreading Awareness And Advocacy

Stigma Surrounding Hepatitis: Breaking The Silence

Even though hepatitis is a common and often treatable illness, the stigma surrounding it is quite strong. Misconceptions regarding the disease's transmission and a lack of knowledge about its prevention and treatment are the causes of this stigma. Because of these misconceptions, people who have hepatitis—whether it is hepatitis B, hepatitis C, or another type—frequently experience prejudice and discrimination.

The stigmatization of hepatitis is mostly due to the connection between the illness and vices including drug abuse and promiscuity. Because of this connection, people who are sick face guilt and shame, which isolates them even more and deters them from getting assistance or telling others they are infected.

Empathy and education are necessary to reduce the stigma associated with hepatitis. We can work to dispel the stigma attached to the illness by presenting factual facts about how hepatitis is spread and highlighting the fact that anybody may get infected, regardless of lifestyle choices. It's critical to stress that anybody, regardless of age, gender, or socioeconomic background, may get hepatitis.

Furthermore, hepatitis may be made to seem less stigmatizing by telling the tales of those who have survived the illness and are living happy, fulfilled lives. Encouraging people to be tested and get treatment for hepatitis may help empower individuals who are infected by highlighting the availability of effective drugs and great treatment results.

Public Health Initiatives And Advocacy Efforts

Advocating for legislation that promotes the prevention, testing, and treatment of hepatitis is a critical function of public health programs. Governmental entities, healthcare professionals, community organizations, and advocacy groups work together on these efforts to adopt solutions that target different facets of hepatitis prevention and control.

A vital element of public health campaigns is advocating for hepatitis B vaccination. Vaccination programs are designed to target high-risk groups, including healthcare professionals, people with certain medical illnesses, people who lead high-risk lifestyles, and newborns born to mothers who have hepatitis B.

Furthermore, public health initiatives concentrate on expanding hepatitis testing and treatment accessibility, especially for marginalized groups who can encounter obstacles in accessing healthcare. This entails carrying out outreach initiatives, offering community health centers free or inexpensive testing, and increasing the availability of reasonably priced prescription drugs.

Additionally, regulations about the prevention and treatment of hepatitis are significantly shaped by advocacy initiatives. Advocates try to educate decision-makers about the effects of hepatitis on public health and the need for financing and resources to support initiatives for prevention and treatment. Additionally, they support laws that guarantee everyone, regardless of financial situation, has access to healthcare services, including hepatitis screening and treatment.

Your Role In Hepatitis Awareness And Prevention

Each of us has a personal responsibility to convey knowledge about hepatitis and stop its spread. Educating ourselves and others on the risk factors, transmission mechanism, and significance of hepatitis testing and treatment is among the most critical things we can do.

We can lower the chance of infection and safeguard others by encouraging healthy habits including having safe sexual relations, not sharing needles or other drug paraphernalia, and receiving the hepatitis B vaccination.

We may also assist groups and campaigns that aim to increase hepatitis awareness and provide assistance and resources to those afflicted with the illness. This might be giving back to the community, taking part in fundraising activities, or just educating our friends, family, and neighbors about hepatitis.

We can have a significant impact on the battle against hepatitis by banding together to end the stigma associated with the disease, supporting laws that encourage prevention and treatment, and taking precautions to keep ourselves and others safe.

CONCLUSION

Hepatitis is a class of viral illnesses that inflame the liver and provide a complicated and diverse global health burden. The study's conclusion on hepatitis covers developments as well as continuous difficulties with the illness's management, prevention, and treatment.

Understanding the several hepatitis viruses, their means of transmission, and the creation of potent vaccinations have advanced significantly in the last few decades. Immunization campaigns, especially those targeting hepatitis B, have been essential in lowering the disease's mortality toll, stopping the spread of new infections, and eventually saving lives.

Furthermore, the therapeutic landscape has changed due to breakthroughs in antiviral medication, providing hope to those with chronic hepatitis infections. Hepatitis C treatment has changed dramatically as a result of direct-acting antivirals (DAAs), which have low side effects and excellent cure rates. These discoveries have not only enhanced clinical results but also decreased the likelihood of liver problems such as hepatocellular carcinoma and cirrhosis.

Nevertheless, there are still a lot of important obstacles to overcome. Many regions of the globe still lack adequate access to reasonably priced medical care, treatment, and diagnostics, especially in low- and middle-income nations. Hepatitis-related stigma and prejudice still impede attempts to spread knowledge, encourage testing, and provide assistance to those who are afflicted.

In addition, constant observation and investigation are necessary due to the advent of novel hepatitis strains and the changing terrain of viral hepatitis. The development of a hepatitis C vaccine and the enhancement of current hepatitis B medicines are ongoing initiatives that need continued funding and cooperation.

In conclusion, despite recent advancements in the battle against hepatitis, sustained efforts are required to resolve lingering issues and meet the World Health Organization's 2030 target of completely eradicating viral hepatitis as a hazard to public health. This calls for a comprehensive strategy that includes support services, treatment, screening, and vaccinations in addition to a dedication to social justice and fairness in the provision of healthcare.

THE END

www.ingramcontent.com/pod-product-compliance
Lightning Source LLC
Chambersburg PA
CBHW051907250726
48659CB00002B/518